A Simple Guide for
MENTAL WELLBEING

(Based on cases commonly seen in Psychiatry Clinic)

Dr. Padmalakshmi Navaneethakrishnan

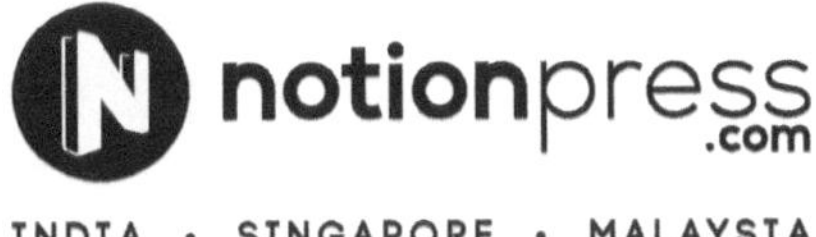

Notion Press Media Pvt Ltd

No. 50, Chettiyar Agaram Main Road,
Vanagaram, Chennai, Tamil Nadu - 600 095

First Published by Notion Press 2021
Copyright © Dr. Padmalakshmi Navaneethakrishnan 2021
All Rights Reserved.

ISBN 978-1-63850-909-7

To my husband Dr. Anbazhahan Rajaram and

my son Dr. Ravisankar Anbazhahan

for their love and support.

CONTENTS

Contents

PREFACE

"An unhealthy mind even in a healthy body will ultimately destroy health."

– Manly Hall

"Mind health" means having a balanced mental and emotional state. This healthy state of mind allows a person to be productive during their day and helps to contribute meaningfully to the community they live in. It is wise to understand this aspect of health to live a successful and purposeful life.

The purpose of this book is to provide an easy guide to common problems that people come across. I have tried to explain using the common cases seen in the outpatient department.

In all these case scenarios, psychiatric treatment is available in the form of tablets, psychotherapy or talking therapy and other lifestyle changes, etc.

This book is not a replacement for consulting a psychiatrist in person. It is only to prompt people to identify the issues, analyse them, and to access professional help appropriately.

Knowledge in mental health aspects may help in mitigating issues arising due to problems like exam failures, death, divorce and domestic violence, etc.

In several families, we come across people with odd behaviour. People normally presume that it is their nature, character or personality and ask everyone around to tolerate and put up with it. Also, people assume that nothing could be done about it. It is not true. This book aims at helping the families to identify those people with troublesome behaviours and seek help from the professionals like psychologists and psychiatrists.

– Dr. N. Padmalakshmi

Description Of The
Icons / Images Used On The Cover:

- These are the components of Mental Well being explained in the book.
- Physical, Mental, Spiritual and Social aspects are represented

 - A happy face – resulting from mental well being

Root (hidden) – identifying the root cause of stress helps in solving it. This is the basis of cognitive behavioural therapy (cbt) 

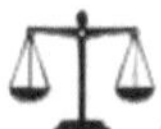 Indicates a balanced state of mind

Meditation helps to get a clear mind. 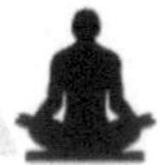

 A loving caring support network – friends / family

A dove - a symbol for peace / compromise 

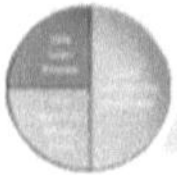 A balanced diet is the fundamental need for A healthy mind and body.

Daily exercise helps in stress reduction and Good physical & mental health 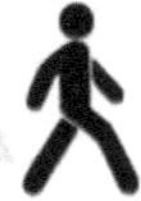

INTRODUCTION

Nowadays, people readily consult psychiatrist for any mental illnesses, unlike the past. Many people suffer from depression at some point in their life. Prevention or early interventions is good for both the patient and the family. This book will help in identifying the factors leading up to a mental health breakdown.

A simple language has been used in this book in order to help even a common man to understand the concepts explained in this book.

If the mental illnesses can be identified at an early stage, the outcome of the disease will be much better. Cure rate will be higher.

This book benefits people in all walks of life like students, singles and feeling lonely, married couples, parents raising kids, women either at home or at work, people going through stresses like job loss, relationship issues, death of loved ones, people with addiction like smoking, drug abuse and alcohol abuse. People with suicidal thoughts and restless behaviours, people with anger problems, comfort eating habits, people with poor sleep, epilepsy and memory loss.

I hope this information will be helpful to you in your everyday life.

CHAPTER 1

8 TIPS FOR BETTER SLEEP

Example Case 1: A young lady believes that her nose is deformed, but her nose looks acceptable to others. She wants to get it operated on by a plastic surgeon. Due to this she could not sleep peacefully at night.

Management of this case: This condition is called *dysmorphophobia*. The treatment could be talk therapy and necessary drugs. There is no need for surgery. Simple understanding of her condition gave her a peace of mind and patient was able to sleep better.

Example Case 2: A 64-year-old lady feels anxious and worried and has a poor sleep. She is afraid of death and unable to cope with life.

Management of this case: This can be a mix of anxiety and depressive disorder. Treatment is counselling, drugs, and ensuring a supportive family environment. Educating them about healthy coping skills will be valuable for them.

Adequate sleep is essential in keeping us happy and healthy. Sleep time is the time at which our body and mind heal itself. Nearly one-third of the world's population has a poor sleep. This condition is called *insomnia*. Typically, adults need 6-8 hours of sleep at night, whereas children need to sleep longer. The measure of the quality of sleep is feeling refreshed in the morning when you wake up.

Here are 8 tips to sleep better at night.

Tip 1: Diet

Eat a balanced healthy diet three times a day. Half the portion should be fibre – either fruits or vegetables. A quarter of the amount should be protein like lentils, eggs or meat. The remaining quarter should be carbohydrates like rice, chapatti, oats, potato or bread. Eat these in moderation. Balanced food keeps your blood sugar levels steady all through the night, and you won't feel hungry in between.

How better can you eat today?

Tip 2: Exercise

You can do any kind of exercise that suits you at a convenient time. Even simple walking for a minimum of 10-30 minutes/day is good enough depending on your fitness level. Avoid vigorous exercise before sleep.

How much exercise did you do today?

Tip 3: Meditation

It is a simple technique involving chanting a mantra, focusing on breathing or mindfulness. Meditation to the mind is what physical exercise is to the body. You should meditate for a minimum of 10-30 minutes a day. It clears the mind, making it emotionally calm and stable.

Have you done your meditation for today?

Tip 4: Sleep environment

Your bedroom should be clean without clutter. It should be well-ventilated, and the room temperature should be comfortable. If lighting is needed, it should be dull and pleasant. Avoid watching television or using mobile phones late at night. Sometimes sleep can be disturbed because of an uncomfortable mattress or pillow. Please check it out.

What changes can you make in your bedroom today?

Tip 5: Bedtime routine

Try to follow some regularity in bedtime because that will support the biological clock in the body. Some people find it useful to have a warm shower, listening to pleasant music, drinking a glass of warm milk, or saying prayers before going to bed.

See which one suits you.

What is your bedtime routine?

Tip 6: Drugs

About 1 or 2 cups of coffee or tea per day are okay. Having too much caffeine makes you alert and interferes with your sleep. Some of the drugs which you are on regularly can also interfere with your sleep. Please check with your doctor.

Are you drinking too much coffee?

Tip 7: Diseases

Some of the diseases are known to cause sleep disturbances—for example, Diabetes, Thyroid illness or depression. If a sleep problem persists, you have to consult your doctor and get it treated.

Is there an illness affecting your sleep?

Tip 8: Resolving Stress

Stress from any physical or mental disorder can affect one's life 24/7 and there by affect sleep. Do not keep accumulating stresses or leave them unattended for a very long time. Try and resolve the issues as soon as possible. Every day before going to bed resolve the stressful issues if possible, by discussing with friends and family.

I hope these tips will help you get a better sleep.

CHAPTER 2

ALCHOHOL ABUSE AND ALCHOHOLISM - HOW TO DEAL WITH IT?

Example Case 3: A middle-aged man who just came out of an alcohol de-addiction centre and relapses into heavy drinking once again because of peer pressure and various stresses in life.

Management of this case: People discharged from de-addiction centres usually need continued support in the form of regular relapse prevention counselling and a supportive environment. In this case, outpatient treatment may not work. He needs readmission and active treatment with appropriate medications. In extreme cases, even change in surroundings like moving home or change in the job, etc. might be needed for long-term recovery.

What is Alcohol?

Alcohol is ethanol. The process of making alcohol is called fermentation, where yeast breaks down sugars in the absence of oxygen. It is used as an ingredient in medicine, cooking, and also as a recreational drug. When consumed, alcohol depresses the central nervous system in the human body. Although, alcohol does not have any nutritional value, some of the drinks do have very high calories which are injurious to health.

Alcoholism is the biggest concern in the current global overview because it is the third leading cause of preventable death and disability, after tobacco and obesity. The incidence of smoking cigarettes is more in drinkers, which adds to the ill effects.

People drink for various reasons.

It is mainly because of stress. Stress can be due to work, family issues, or financial issues.

Also, people drink when they are happy while partying and celebrating.

Teenagers usually drink due to curiosity and peer pressure. Easy availability of alcohol is an important cause. In some cultures, alcohol is an integral part of the daily routine. Finally, we should not forget the genetic vulnerability of an individual, which is also a cause of alcoholism.

When we consume alcohol, the immediate effects can be elated mood, loss of inhibition, poor coordination and balance, slurred speech, vomiting, and behavioural changes. Due to excess drinking, people might become unconscious and can even die.

When people continue drinking for a very long time, every organ in the body gets affected. For example – in the liver, it causes cirrhosis, in the heart, it causes weakness, in the stomach, it causes ulcers and even cancer.

Due to their behavioural changes, the alcoholics might even lose their job. Domestic violence is a major issue created by drinkers. Also, they will get involved in crimes, robbery, and drunken driving.

There are three stages of drinking – early, middle and late stages.

It is crucial to know these stages clearly because this is what is going to help us to identify the safe and unsafe range of drinking alcohol.

The three stages are:

In Stage 1 – which is an experimental stage, people drink for social reasons. Occasionally they binge drink also. Without binge drinking, just less frequent social drinking is fine. But beyond this stage, caution and intervention are needed.

In Stage 2 – which is the middle stage, alcohol is abused. They drink more frequently and in secret. They drink to avoid withdrawal symptoms.

In Stage 3 – which is late or the end-stage, there is alcohol dependence. People lose control over drinking. Their life revolves only around alcohol. Despite physical and mental health problems, they keep drinking. They lose precious things in life like relationships, jobs, etc.

Unfortunately, many people and their families are suffering without proper help. Hence, awareness about the problem and the available treatment needs to be discussed widely on various platforms. Usually, patients get admitted to the hospital only when they encounter issues like fits, tremors, hearing voices when alone, jaundice, or stomach pain.

Ideally, help should be sought voluntarily by the patient or helped by the relatives based on the stages of drinking.

How to deal with it?

Nowadays, excellent treatment facilities are available for people who have problems with drinking. If you consult any doctor, he will guide you to the right de-addiction centre after doing preliminary investigations.

De-addiction centres have an expert medical team that will help stop drinking by constant supervision and by providing necessary medications and support. Outpatient detoxification is also available. Benzodiazepines like chlordiazepoxide and vitamin B1 called Thiamine form an essential part of drug regimen in the treatment of this condition. In the long run, the onus is on the individual to quit alcohol. He can get help from family, friends, psychiatrists, or even psychologists as needed. There is an internationally established organization like Alcoholics Anonymous. These are self-help groups, and they have changed the lives of many.

CHAPTER 3
SUICIDAL THOUGHTS - HOW TO HANDLE IT?

Example Case 4: A middle-aged woman feeling suicidal and hearing voices when alone – telling her to kill herself. She stops eating and drinking. She stops talking to others.

Management of this case: This is severe depression with psychosis which certainly needs a psychiatrist's intervention. The recovery rate is very good.

Suicide is an act of intentionally killing oneself. Worldwide every year, almost 900,000 people die by committing suicide, i.e., approximately one death every 40 seconds. Suicide is the second leading cause of death in the world in the age group of 15-24 years. Depression is the leading cause of this disability around the globe.

Message for people with suicidal thoughts:

✦ Do not feel lonely – try and reach out for help – you are not alone.

✦ Do not give up hope – life is precious and worth living.

✦ Do not feel helpless – there are several solutions to the same problem. Help is available. Get professional help if necessary.

✦ Do not think you are a burden to others – talk through and find out what others feel about you?

✦ Please check if you are depressed – in this case, you may not know there is a future.

✦ Do not hesitate. Ring suicide prevention helpline. They are available for you 24x7.

✦ If you are facing a financial crisis – seek the right financial advice personally for you.

✦ Please, don't give up on life!

✦ Do not be impulsive or aggressive.

✦ Do not jump to conclusions – try and find the truth.

✦ Life is adventurous and full of challenges.

Life is too short, anyway. In short, people with depression have negative thoughts and they feel lonely, helpless and hopeless. They feel life is not worth living and that there is no future for them.

The reality may not be that bad after all. That is why, it will be helpful for them if they talk to a doctor and go through the right treatment process by which they can get over suicidal thoughts.

Management:

1. Depression can be treated using SSRI, TCA, or SNRI group of antidepressant drugs.

2. In addition, CBT also helps.

CHAPTER 4

SLEEPING PILL ADDICTION AND WAYS TO COME OFF SLEEPING PILLS

Example Case 5: A middle-aged man gets prescribed sleeping pills for treatment of poor sleep. He continues to use this prescription for several years and buys the same medicines without going for psychiatric consultation and review. That medicine stops working, and he has nights of poor sleep.

Management of this case: This is a sleeping pill addiction. The underlying cause of sleep disorder needs to be investigated and treated. This will help to come off sleeping pills gradually.

Each year millions of individuals use sleeping pills to achieve, longer and better sleep cycles every night. Core or essential part of sleep is just 3-4 hours/night; hence, 6-8 hours of sleep is adequate for adults. Older people need less sleep. Feeling refreshed while awake is the target. Studies have proved that in normal sleep, the concept of catch-up sleep does not work. Adequate sleep is needed every day.

What is insomnia?

Insomnia is sleeping less than 6 hours/night either due to delay in falling asleep or waking up early. You feel tired when waking up. Benzodiazepines like nitrazepam and Z-group drugs like Zolpidem or Zopiclone, are commonly used. These are used to treat insomnia and should be taken only for 1-2 weeks.

Over the counter, drugs like herbal products are not clinically proven to help sleep and can cause organ damage.

Tips for safer use of sleeping pills:

+ Avoid frequent use.
+ Take it only when you have enough time of at least 7-8 hours of sleep.
+ Never drive a car or operate machinery after taking the pill.
+ Never mix it with alcohol.

Risks and side effects of sleeping tablets:

It can cause drowsiness, confusion, dementia and falls. People may need higher doses over time. Addiction to the drug can result in an intense craving for the drug. You are likely to be dependent on the medication. It can lead to withdrawal symptoms like rebound insomnia, depression, anxiety-like tremor, and palpitation. It can begin in a few hours to a few days and lasts up to 1-2 weeks.

Drug overdose:

It can cause permanent brain damage. It can also lead to excess lethargy, drunk-like behaviour, abdominal pain, and breathing irregularities. This is called prescription drug misuse. Therefore, it is not a good idea to buy these medicines in bulk.

What is the alternative for better sleep?

1. Healthy habits – not pills.

2. Avoid daytime naps.

3. Treat physical and mental health problems, which are likely to cause insomnia. Consult your doctor.

4. Cognitive Behavioural Therapy (CBT) is the most powerful tool for better sleep, which helps in identifying negative thoughts,

emotions, and behaviour. It is proven to be helpful especially in case of depression and insomnia. Good thoughts and actions are a part of CBT.

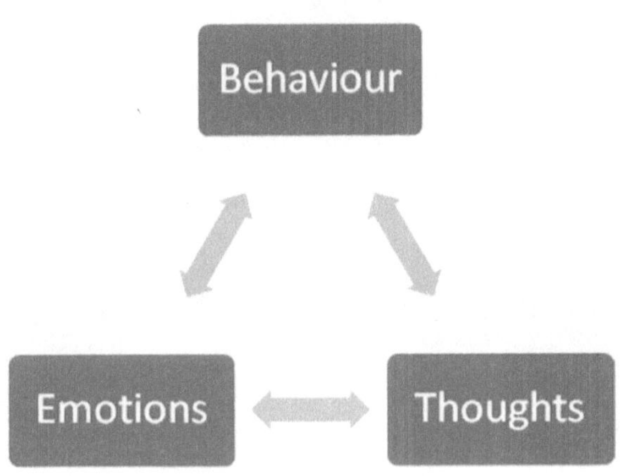

5. Have a healthy balanced diet – 50% fibre, 25% protein, 25% carbohydrate in each plate of food.

6. Regular exercise can be done at any time for at least 30 minutes per day.

7. Exposure to fresh air helps to sleep better. It is a powerful sleep aid.

8. Practice meditation for at least 20-30 minutes/day. It can help in the healing of some physical and psychiatric ailments also.

How to manage sleeping pill addiction?

Medical supervision is needed to come off the sleeping pills in a step-by-step manner. Counselling helps too.

CHAPTER 5

LONELINESS AND EIGHT TIPS FOR WHAT YOU CAN DO ABOUT IT

Example Case 6: A middle-aged man wandering the streets with poor self-care, dirty clothes, and hears voices and speaks to himself when alone, over a long period. His sleep is disturbed.

Management of this case: This condition is likely to be Schizophrenia for which excellent drugs are available. In the long term, such people can be helped by monitoring drug compliance and reuniting them with their families when they recover from their mental illness.

Man is a social animal, which means that being connected to people around you is an essential component of happy living. In case you do not have enough meaningful relationships, then you will feel a negative, painful emotion and this is called loneliness. It is a common human emotion; however, the degree of the loneliness felt varies with each individual. I will suggest some practical ways to get over this issue.

"Chronic loneliness" is a term used to describe loneliness that lasts over a more extended period. It is not a specific mental health condition. It has now become a paramount public health concern as millions of men and women are affected by it worldwide.

A study showed that the age group of 16-24 years was feeling lonelier than the over-65 years age group of people. On the bright side, loneliness is treatable.

Loneliness Vs. Solitude:

Loneliness gives a negative feeling, while solitude gives a positive feeling. Solitude is being alone voluntarily for self-reflection, contemplation, meditation, creativity, self-growth, and self-realization.

Causes of loneliness:

1. *Situational loneliness* – due to divorce, death, increased life expectancy especially in females, change of schools, job, work from home, or moving to a new city.

2. *Developmental loneliness* – due to family separation, physical, or psychological disability.

3. *Internal loneliness* – mental illness, a feeling of low self-worth and low self-esteem, or living alone for the first time.

Warning signs:

Warning signs to look out for include getting sick frequently, body aches and pains, low energy, poor sleep and appetite, anxiety and restless, feeling of self-doubt, hopelessness, worthlessness, and inability to focus.

Problems of loneliness:

It has adverse effects on both physical and mental health. Increased stress leads to a higher risk of cardiovascular disease and stroke. You become more prone to drug and alcohol use which in turn can lead to antisocial behaviour. It can cause memory problems, and poor decision-making. There is an increased risk of depression which can then lead to social withdrawal behaviour and more likelihood of suicide.

What can you do about it?

1. Identify and get your physical and mental health issues treated.

2. If you can go out physically, go to parks, clubs, or any social gatherings.

3. Make regular visits to places of worship like churches, mosques, or temples.

4. Trace the family tree or good old school friends - this can bring interesting personalities back into your life.

5. Develop a hobby and find people with similar interests.

6. Volunteer for community activities - it is a noble and effective method that can be fulfilling.

7. With current technology using phones and the internet, you can communicate via social media like WhatsApp, Facebook, Instagram and Twitter.

8. Join virtual groups/clubs like self-help groups, helplines, etc.

Take home message:

The moment you start feeling lonely, it is the time for action. So far, we discussed several ways and means of dealing with it.

What action are you going to take to make you feel connected with the society again?

CHAPTER 6

PARENTING SKILLS - 12 TIPS

Example Case 7: A smart boy in school performing well in extracurricular activities like sports, music, arts and crafts and fails miserably in his studies.

Management of this case: Assess his IQ first. Your doctor would like to conduct some blood tests to identify the cause for his poor performance in school. If it is normal, then career selection should be guided based on *his* interests and capabilities. Psychometric analysis can also be used to identify his strengths.

The style of parenting is one of the most researched fields in psychology. There is no one-size-fits-all strategy to it. Every child is unique. Depending on the surroundings and bringing up, he/she becomes either a good or a bad individual.

So, parents play a significant role in providing the right environment.

Tip 1: Unconditional love

Apart from providing essentials like food, clothing and shelter, the most crucial component is the unconditional love that you show to your kids. Also, a healthy relationship with your spouse will benefit in having a positive effect on your children's behaviour. Children from low-conflict families are happier and turn out to be more successful.

Tip 2: A strong sense of security

Children who get a strong sense of security early on perform better later.

Tip 3: Quality time

Make sure you spend one-on-one quality time with your children; however, busy you are - this should be a priority in your life. Make time to talk every day even about non-school related topics like sharing your life experiences and your interests. Engage in activities with them like homework, games, storytelling, or even doing fun activities. It helps in building a good relationship with your child. Parents not understanding the significance of spending quality time with their kids - is one of the top reasons for the poor development of a child's personality.

Tip 4: Listen to what your kids say

Help your children to express themselves by encouraging them to talk freely. Put yourself in their shoes and try to understand *their* point of view - this is called *empathy*. Apart from listening to their words, observe their body language, and understand their emotions completely. Involve them in decision making whenever possible. Better communication is the key to a better style of parenting.

Tip 5: Disciplining

A set of rules and boundaries regarding bedtime, mealtime, study time and playtime. Also give your children responsibilities, like doing chores around the house. These are essential life skills, which no one else will teach. Follow a warm and firm parenting style with your disciplining. Time out technique is also useful.

Tip 6: Be a good role model

Being a good role model is the way to teach how children should behave. For example, if you drink or smoke, then it will not be appropriate if you tell your children not to drink or smoke drugs.

Tip 7: No physical or mental abuse, no matter what

Never hit them or shout at them. Avoid shaming in front of others as it would hurt their ego. Avoid belittling them by comparing them with others because every child is unique and talented. They can shine if we help in honing their skills and provide them the right opportunity.

Tip 8: Reward good behaviour

It is a positive reinforcement which can be done by verbal appreciation, using a star chart or by giving food treats, etc. It is an effective strategy.

Tip 9: Quality relations and social skills

Mentor your children and highlight the significance of having a quality circle of loving friends and relatives. Teach them to focus on the needs of others as well. This social network is like a safety net, which can safeguard them when they are about to tip over. Children empowered with social skills are more self-confident and become successful adults. Also, teach them moral values like sharing, accepting the differences, disagreeing *respectfully*, being polite and complimenting others, and asking for help in the right manner at the right time.

Tip 10: Dealing with unhappiness

Adverse events like failure in exams, being dumped by a lover, death of a loved one, etc. will evoke stronger negative emotions. Teach your children facing such challenges positively as it is one of the essential skills to become successful. It is rightly said - *When the going gets tough, the tough get going.* Train them to be resilient and keep going. Guide them about what is under their control and what is not. Educate them that while facing difficulties in life, resolving to extreme measures like drugs or suicide is not the right option. Let them know that trust in the supreme power or God helps us when things are not under our control. Once the children sense a supportive environment, they will ask for help. It is the parent's responsibility to create such an environment.

Tip 11: Career guidance

While selecting higher education or job, help them in identifying their capabilities and interests and facilitate them in choosing the right path. Online Psychometric tests could be used as a tool to provide useful insights.

Tip 12: Be human

No human being is perfect, including yourself. Remember how you grew up. Do not expect your children to be an imitation of you or someone else. Give allowance for making mistakes.

Follow the above tips gently, customize it according to the children's needs and let them know that you have complete faith in them. Give them enough space, and you will notice them blossoming into a beautiful flower – much more beautiful than what you expect of them.

I hope these tips are useful to parents who have kids of all age groups.

CHAPTER 7

RESTLESSNESS AND ITS MANAGEMENT

Case 8: A middle-aged man who is full of energy, over-talkative with pressure of speech and behaves in a disinhibited manner with ladies. He wastes money by overspending and being careless, which lasts for a week or more. Then he has mood swings, and suddenly he becomes sorrowful, which lasts for at least two weeks or more. He also has tiredness, lack of interest in activities and sleeplessness.

Answer: This condition is "Manic depressive psychosis or bipolar disorder" when this happens repeatedly. This condition needs mood stabilizers and regular monitoring.

Case 9: A young adult abuses illicit street drugs and feels high in the mood. He starts hearing voices when alone. He feels suspicious that people are trying to kill him or trying to spy on him.

Answer: Drug-induced psychosis which can be treated with medicines and by stopping illicit drug abuse.

Case 10: A young adult believes that someone has done black magic on him, and he is unable to sleep.

Answer: This is possibly acute transient psychosis. This can be treated with appropriate drugs, including sleeping pills if necessary. Educating them about tips for better sleep will be helpful also.

Feeling restless is usually a sign of anxiety or agitation. It is a behaviour where people are fidgety, pacing up and down, and unable to relax.

Motor restlessness is the compelling urge to move and the inability to sit still. When anxious, they can be worried all the time, muscles of their body are stiff when tense, and they feel on edge all the time. These symptoms are troublesome when these affect your day-to-day life routine, work, sleep or appetite.

In the case of drug or alcohol abuse, there is restless behaviour, and they commit petty crimes to fund their drug abuse.

In bipolar disorder, as part of the manic episode, they feel elated in mood which lasts for a week at least, they waste money, they have more energy and sleep only for a few hours, and they can be restless.

Depressed or anxious personality disorder patients are always nervous, and it is difficult to treat.

In Schizophrenia, there may be wandering behaviour because of this restlessness.

Old age people with dementia will also encounter memory problems.

Management:

1. Physical exercise and stretches for relieving muscle tension.

2. Meditation for calming the mind.

3. Deep breathing exercises to relieve anxiety.

4. Treat underlying depression and anxiety with medications.

5. Treat dementia, Schizophrenia, and Bipolar disorder with medications.

6. Treat drug and alcohol abuse with detoxification therapy.

If all these underlying conditions are left untreated, there is a risk of suicide in these patients.

CHAPTER 8

ANGER AND DOMESTIC VIOLENCE - HOW TO DEAL WITH IT?

Case 11: A middle-aged man in a full-time job feels suspicious about his wife's fidelity and believes that she is having an affair. He is an alcoholic. He ends up beating his wife without any reason. He hires a man to monitor his wife's behaviour secretly by following her.

Answer: This condition is "paranoid delusion", and it can be corrected by controlling alcohol dependence with the help of de-addiction centres as alcohol usage can worsen this condition. Drugs play an important role in curing this condition.

Anger is a normal and even healthy emotion, but it is essential to deal with it appropriately. Uncontrolled anger can take a toll on both your health and your relationships.

What is domestic violence?

It broadly includes all acts of physical, sexual, psychological or economic violence that may be committed by a family member or an intimate partner. Domestic violence can cause physical and emotional harm to children and young people in the household.

Warning signs of violence are:

+ Loss of temper daily

+ Frequent physical fighting

+ Property damage

+ Use of drugs or alcohol

+ Plans to commit acts of violence

People under abuse are more likely to develop anxiety, depression, substance abuse and thoughts of suicide. Domestic violence makes up 21% of all violent crimes. Managing anger problems and issues of domestic violence is important for a stable marriage.

How to deal with it?

1. Decide to control anger and avoid violence.

2. Breathe deeply and count from 1-10, when you feel you are angry.

3. Slowly repeat "relax" or "take it easy" till your anger subsides.

4. Walk away from the situation.

5. Avoid alcohol or illicit drugs that can make you more likely to act on angry feelings impulsively and commit acts of violence.

6. If you are physically injured, do not hesitate to get help – neighbours, helplines, ambulance, or police as appropriate

7.   Important point to consider is that anger or irritable mood can be a symptom of underlying depression. Please consult your doctor.

CHAPTER 9

STRESS - HEALTHY AND UNHEALTHY COPING SKILLS

Case 12: A middle-aged woman eats lots of junk food for comfort as a way of coping with stress and ends up being obese with a lot of other physical health problems. She does not do exercise.

Answer: This is likely to be a binge eating disorder which can be managed by treating underlying depression. Cognitive behavioural therapy, drugs and lifestyle modifications like exercise and healthy eating are the modalities of treatment. Educating them about healthy coping skills will also be beneficial in the long term.

Stressful situations in life can test our strength. When stressed, stress hormones like adrenaline and cortisol are released, and there is a fight or flight response in the body that causes increased heart rate and rapid breathing. Highest level of stress comes from life events like the death of a loved one or spouse and other life events like divorce, moving to a new house, loss of job, severe injury, or illness, etc. Each individual has different ways of coping with stress and have varying levels of tolerance. So, it is not only the nature of the event, causing the pressure but the individual's ability to accept, adjust and come to terms with these life changes that matter.

Long term stress can affect a person from head to foot:

+ *In the brain*: It causes tension headache, poor sleep, anxiety, depression and increased risk of stroke.

+ *In the chest*: It worsens asthma, risk of heart attack.

+ *In the abdomen:* Acid reflux or heartburn, diarrhoea, constipation, risk of developing type 2 diabetes.

Healthy and unhealthy coping skills is a matter of personal choice.

First, let us look at unhealthy coping skills. It worsens stress and does not solve the problems. They are done just to relieve tension. Some examples are self-harm by cutting their arms, comfort eating, damaging material things, taking to drug and alcohol abuse.

On the other hand, healthy coping skills distract your mind and engage you in creative activities that will help you get rid of stress and negative thoughts.

A few healthy coping skills have been mentioned below:

1. *Having a hobby:* It distracts your mind from worries, and you don't mind spending time doing it. Watching television all day is bad for health. Be active. Singing, dancing, gardening, or listening to music improves your mood. Learning musical instruments keeps your brain alert for a long time over the years.

   You can also try painting where you play with colours, arts and crafts – thereby improving your creativity. Reading books is an excellent hobby, like personal development books, joke books and newspapers for general knowledge, etc.

   If a person is losing interest in hobbies, it is called Anhedonia, which is a well-known symptom of depression.

2. *Writing down in a notebook:* It helps in processing and clarifying your thoughts. Use it as an emotional outlet for your feelings.

It is a kind of expression similar to talking to someone. It helps in releasing pent up emotions. It is immensely beneficial for the person who is doing it.

An extra tip – you can maintain a food or diet chart, sleep chart, mood, or activity chart – depending on your needs to monitor your progress. An important fact is that the expression of emotion is affected in severe depression.

3. *Talking to someone:* Helps to let out the pent-up emotions, thereby leads to problem-solving. Although, friends and family can be supportive, professional help can be more therapeutic. Also, an empathetic listening is needed. Social isolation has an association with depression. Do not underestimate the power of talking things through. It can change your life for good. During counselling, someone listens to you, and they help you to find solutions which are best suited for you. The more experienced the therapist, the better is the outcome.

4. *Exercise:* Walking is proven to uplift your mood during depression. Exercise releases happy hormones. Motivation to exercise every day can come from yourself or the people around you. There are many people who form groups for running, badminton, etc. Do try out

yoga, gym workout or meditation. Get trained on how to do it the right way. In depression, people get tired quickly and do not exercise.

5. *Developing a sense of humour:* A person must make a habit of laughing for simple joys in life with others, but not "at" others. He/she can share a joke often and work on developing that skill. It is a healthy coping mechanism.

6. *Go on a holiday:* A day's tour or a planned vacation to a new environment can refresh you.

7. *Pamper yourself:* You can pamper yourself by taking massages, which can rejuvenate you. Try to do it regularly, once in a month or whenever you feel overwhelmed.

8. *Going for shopping:* Going for shopping can be pleasurable. It need not be an expensive venture.

9. *Opt for spiritual practices:* If you are willing, you can opt for spiritual practices like chanting, prayers, or rituals regularly. For many it helps in cleansing the cluttered mind.

In essence, by doing these activities, you can enhance your feel-good factor and live a better-quality life.

What is your personal choice – healthy or unhealthy coping skills?

CHAPTER 10

FITS (EPILEPSY) AND DEPRESSION - ITS MANAGEMENT

Case 13: A young adult with repeated fits or seizures for many years, is feeling low in mood for over two weeks because of limitations in social life and tired all the time. He is unable to drive a car to work.

Answer: This condition is epilepsy with depression. Excellent drugs are available to treat this condition. A fits frequency chart can help monitor the progress.

The risk of deliberate self-harm is greater in patients with fits. Around 50 million people worldwide have epilepsy making it one of the most common neurological diseases globally. Nearly 80% of people with epilepsy live in low- or middle-income countries. Up to 70% of people living with epilepsy could live seizure-free if diagnosed correctly and treated appropriately.

Fits is a neurological condition that causes seizures. Seizures or fits happens when your brain's electrical activity becomes abnormal. A seizure disorder can occur in head injuries and alcohol withdrawal.

Different types of seizures can occur. The patient might shake violently, lose consciousness and fall to the floor. Within a few minutes, he will be awake but feel sleepy or confused, or he might lose awareness of his surroundings and keep staring for a few seconds.

Patients with epilepsy are more prone to depression and anxiety. They cannot drive a vehicle, and their social life may be limited. In many cases, the cause is unknown.

Causes of depression in epilepsy patients are hormonal imbalance, side effects of anti-seizure drugs, and psychosocial factors like isolation as epilepsy is a long-term medical condition.

What is Depression?

The symptoms of depression are tiredness, low mood and lack of interest in pleasurable activities. When 2 out of 3 symptoms persist for at least two weeks or more, it is called depression. There may or may not be a lot of other associated symptoms affecting sleep, appetite, body weight, memory and concentration. They may be suspicious, hearing voices when alone and feel suicidal when there is severe depression.

What triggers a seizure?

+ Stress or anxiety
+ Some medicines like antidepressants or antipsychotics
+ Lack of sleep or tiredness
+ Irregular meals
+ Heavy alcohol intake or using street drugs
+ Flickering lights example from videogames
+ Menstrual periods
+ High fever

Safety precautions at home, school or workplace in epileptic patients:

1. Replace glass, e.g., glass doors, cups, etc., with plastic to prevent injuries.

2. Avoid swimming alone. Showers are safer than baths.

3. Cooking related activities can be dangerous and result in burns. Do not do it alone.

4. Always keep one door unlocked in the house when you are alone.

5. Use only motorized power tools that have safety switches.

6. Make family and friends aware of your seizures and what they need to do to help you in case of fits.

Investigations:

1. *Electroencephalogram (EEG):* EEG may be useful in diagnosing epilepsy and other seizure disorders. It is a test that detects electrical activity in your brain using small, metal discs attached to your scalp. While monitoring an epileptic patient, a fits chart helps to markdown the frequency. This chart will provide useful information for the treating doctor to monitor progress.

2. *CT Scan/MRI brain:* A CT Scan/MRI brain helps to rule out head injury.

3. *Blood test will help:* For example, Liver function test, especially Gamma-glutamyl transferase – a specific test to identify alcohol abuse. A blood test will help in identifying and treating Anaemia and Hypothyroidism which can also cause depression.

Arriving at the right diagnosis:

A clear description of what happened during the seizure by the person affected and if possible, from an eyewitness, is essential for diagnosis. Only 2 out of 10 people experience fits despite medication. Having a seizure as a one-off incident is not called epilepsy. Having a certain number of fits in a year qualifies for a diagnosis of epilepsy. Eptoin is a commonly used antiepileptic medication. It controls seizures by decreasing the abnormal and excessive activity of nerve cell in the brain.

Management:

Medications help significantly in controlling epilepsy. Antidepressant like bupropion may increase the frequency of seizures. Treating epilepsy and depression at the same time can be a challenge. The best treatment approach is to start low, go slow and use the lowest effective dose of medication.

In addition to medication, lifestyle changes like regular exercise and talking therapy also help. If treated adequately, this condition has good outcome.

If correctly identified and treated, the response to antidepressants for depression is excellent. Cognitive Behavioural therapy also helps.

CHAPTER 11

WHAT TO EAT TO MAKE YOU PHYSICALLY FIT AND MENTALLY HAPPY?

Food is any nutritious substance that we eat or drink to maintain life and growth. A healthy balanced diet can be based on local eating patterns, using locally available foods and respecting eating customs.

Attitude towards food:

Have a balanced mindset where you neither worship nor hate or fear food. People wanting to lose weight have a fear of food. They think they need to be hungry to lose weight. This is a poor understanding of nutrition. Others eat when they are worried or happy.

What not to eat?

Junk food provides empty calories. They have high sugar and salt content with unhealthy fat.

Also, there are no life-sustaining elements like protein, fibre, vitamins and minerals.

For example: Chips, cake, pop drinks, fried savouries, sweets and ice cream. If at all people should have some fear about the food, they should fear these junk foods when taken in excess.

What to eat?

Eat a balanced healthy diet. Eat a variety of fruits and vegetables of all colours. Eat happy foods like dark chocolate, banana, nuts and seeds, oats, fatty fish, probiotic yoghurt, orange, mango, kiwi, strawberry and grapes in moderation.

What is a Fad diet?

It is a diet that is popular for a time like fads in fashion. It is not a standard dietary recommendation.

For example – paleo diet – is a kind of diet based on foods eaten by early humans. The lifestyle of hunters and gatherers is not suited for current times.

How to handle eating out?

No one can avoid eating out altogether. We just need to develop a system to suit our needs.

+ Follow the plate method even in the hotels – especially if you are in a buffet.

+ Take less of deep-fried or greasy items.

+ Try several salads for fibre.

+ For protein, get grilled, barbecued or tandoor non-vegetarian items, mushroom, or paneer.

+ Carbohydrate can be a smaller portion.

+ Take less of sugary desserts and drinks.

CHAPTER 12

WORK-LIFE BALANCE AND COMMON WORK-RELATED ISSUES

Case 14: A middle-aged man with repeated checking of completed files at work, repeated checking of door locks and repeated washing of hands because of repetitive thoughts of dirt and contamination.

Answer: This condition is called "obsessive-compulsive disorder" (OCD). Treatment is with talk therapy and specific drugs. Some patients may need lifelong treatment.

Initially, when people start working at a young age, they will be enthusiastic in earning money and will not mind working overtime. But with increasing age and health issues or family issues, they may not be able to work overtime. They will generally slowdown in pace and take more sick leaves. Maintain a steady pace at work throughout your work life. You need to think about being productive in the long term than just thinking about short term monetary gains. Spending time regularly to maintain physical and mental health is crucial. By doing this, you will feel more energetic and enthusiastic about working for an extended period. Your sick leave will be less. You will get a good reputation, and you will be able to maintain good work relationships also. When your health is right, you will enjoy a quality family time which will then encourage you to get better at work. It is a vicious cycle. There is a saying "work while you work, play while you play".

While you are at work, be entirely focused on work. When you are with family, enjoy relaxation and fun. It is also a good idea to allocate some free personal space for rest and reflection. Ensure you get good quality sleep at night every day.

Also, try to ensure you get paid appropriately for the hours of work that you put in. Try and find a position from where you enjoy working and one that can give you job satisfaction.

Common work-related issues include:

1. *Job loss:* It can be expected or sudden. To prevent this, you should develop your skills

and work to improve your company's profit. Then job loss is less likely. If it happens then take it easy and try a different company. Do not lose hope. Having a degree of financial stability will help to cope with the situation better till you find the next job.

2. *Job transfer:* This can bring additional stress of house move and settling in a new place and making new friends. Sometimes, this can be accompanied by promotion and pay rise that makes things a bit easier to cope. But job promotion also brings additional responsibilities that cannot be avoided and can be challenging to manage.

3. *Problems with the boss and work colleagues:* If you are going to work regularly without taking unnecessary sick leave, your boss will be happy. You should also try to complete projects on time. It is good to be a team player. This way, you can get along well with your colleagues. If there are any issues, you must communicate and get help. If you maintain your physical and mental health, you can cope better. You may need to do extra work to cover for absent colleagues. Please remember that your work will also be covered when you take time off work.

Any of these issues, when not dealt appropriately, can lead to depression because of work-related stress.

Help is available.

Do not hesitate to contact a professional for treatment and support.

CHAPTER 13

MARRIAGE - 12 TIPS TO MAKE IT WORK

Case 15: A middle-aged woman feels suspicious that a camera or postman is spying her. She believes that her husband has poisoned her food.

Answer: This condition is "paranoid delusion". Effective drugs are available now.

Case 16: A middle-aged woman feels worried all the time with aches and pains in the body which do not go away with painkillers.

Answer: *Diagnosis:* Generalized anxiety disorder

Treatment: Drugs, counselling and lifestyle modifications such as breathing exercises and meditation. Family support will also help her.

It is worrisome to investigate the divorce rates in different countries. Recent statistics showing the divorce rates in various countries are as follows: Belarus 68%, Russian Federation 65%, Sweden 64%, Latvia 63%, Ukraine 63%, Czech Republic 61%, US 46%, China 2% and India 1%.

We can clearly see such gross differences in divorce rates based on the cultural values and moral values of the people in different parts of the world.

Please remember that marriage is hard work. It is up to you to make it worthwhile.

The fundamental human values and mindset to make the marriage to work are as follows:

1. Be kind, caring and forgiving towards each other.

2. Share your responsibilities.

3. Communicate your feelings and provide emotional support by listening carefully.

4. Avoid physical violence and mental torture.

5. Do activities together, like cooking and exercise that will improve your bonding.

6. Couples should work towards stabilising their relationship before planning for a baby.

7. Set a conflict resolution time such as avoiding it in the early morning hours or setting it before bedtime if possible.

8. Be appreciative and bring out the best in each other. Couple should try to understand each other's strengths and weaknesses and try to complement each other. One person helping to bring the best out of other person is one of the secrets of creating a strong bond in a relationship.

9. Set certain boundaries to deal with others.

10. Avoid blaming each other if things go wrong.

11. Allocate quiet time for yourself and enjoy your solitude.

12. It is the companionship which sustains a marriage in the long run, rather than the romance which is only short lived.

BEREAVEMENT REACTION

Case 17: An ex-military man having nightmares and flashbacks about a traumatic incident and reliving the past.

Answer: This is a post-traumatic stress disorder (PTSD). This can be treated with drugs and psychotherapy. Lifestyle changes like change of job will also help.

Case 18: A young woman lost her dad suddenly and then starts hearing his voice when alone and thinks he is still alive.

Answer: This is denial as a part of the bereavement reaction. Hearing voices before going to sleep or in the early morning hours is nothing to worry about in this case. It will be helpful to undertake healthy coping strategies. Drugs can be used if necessary. Counselling also helps.

What is bereavement?

It is the state of having lost a relative or close friend who has recently died. Adaptation to such a loss usually takes 6-12 months. The intensity of grief may flare during the death anniversaries of the loved one.

Bereavement reaction can precipitate or worsen some mental disorders like depression, anxiety, post-traumatic stress disorder and alcohol abuse.

What is grief reaction?

It is the natural response following the death of a loved one. The pattern and intensity of grief vary over time as the suffering individual adapts to the loss. Acute grief is intense and short duration.

Symptoms of separation distress are seeking proximity to deceased, crying, loneliness, social withdrawal and disinterest in other people and activities not associated with the dead. They may hear the voices of the deceased when alone.

What is complicated grief?

It is a form of acute grief that is unusually prolonged, intense and disabling and serious psychosocial problems impede adaptation to the loss.

What happens when there is a sudden loss?

Death of a loved one can be intense and painful, regardless of the manner of death. Sudden loss due to illness, violence or accident can produce intense acute grief. They may feel numb and disconnected from the world. Homicide (murder) or suicide can trigger anger or guilt about the death.

Prior psychiatric history, less social support, female gender, severe depression and death of a loved one by suicide, increase the risk of suicidal ideation and behaviour among the bereaved.

Management:

Several rituals are held during and after funeral. They vary according to cultures. Irrespective of the literal meaning of the rituals, performing them along with the near and dear ones helps greatly in bringing inner peace in the bereaved family.

If grief symptoms are unduly prolonged, they may need to be treated for the underlying depression. Do not hesitate to get professional help when necessary.

Chapter 9 describes coping strategies for stress.

15 TIPS FOR STUDYING WELL - HOW TO DEAL WITH EXAM FAILURE?

Unfortunately, exam failures or under performance is one of the major causes of mental distress for the student community. This leads to several suicides or depression among the students around the time of publishing exam results. The students, parents and friends need to be aware of this issue and be informed about how to face such situations.

Here are 15 tips for it:

1. Be self-disciplined.

2. Have a regular study time.

3. Eat a healthy balanced diet.

4. Take regular breaks like watching television or going for a walk.

5. Sleep well – good quality sleep helps to consolidate the learnt study material.

6. Have self-confidence.

7. Have a recreational activity like singing, dancing, or sports.

8. Work using a timetable planned for exams.

9. Focus on your study technique - like taking notes, underlining keywords, using flashcards, etc.

10. Be regular in attendance at school or college.

11. Good time management – make sure you have enough time to revise before exams.

12. Meditation helps to focus on studies.

13. *Psychometric Analysis:* This is a test to analyse the ability and personality of a student to take up a particular subject for higher studies and career. Just liking a subject or just guided by a relative should not be the way to a career path. These tests are available online and utilising these scientific methods will ensure the higher performance of the students in that chosen field.

14. *Career Guidance Counsellors:* They do a good job of assessing the student's capacity, assessing the educational courses available and guiding the students accordingly.

15. *Mentors: They* are experienced, wise and trusted teachers who guide the students

during the course. Some schools and colleges officially allot a mentor. If not, students can approach any good teacher.

People with suicidal thoughts, please refer to chapter 3 for detailed explanation on how to handle it.

Please remember, "Failures are the stepping stones to success." When guided properly, students have a lot of learning and self-growth. This makes it an enjoyable phase in life for many.

CHAPTER 16
WOMEN'S HEALTH

Case 19: A middle-aged woman gets irritable a few days before menstrual periods and feels bloated and tearful. It happens every month, and she feels better after the start of menses.

Answer: This is premenstrual syndrome or tension, which is treated with regular exercise, drinking plenty of water and eating a healthy diet and a few specific drugs. Generally, it is a self-limiting common condition.

> **Case 20:** A 30-year-old woman delivers a baby, and then after a few days, she feels low in mood and unable to take care of the baby. She is tired and has a poor sleep which lasts at least for two weeks.
>
> **Answer:** This is post-natal depression. It is different from "post-natal blues", which means feeling low in the mood just for a few days, which goes off by itself. Psychiatrist involvement is essential in such cases.

Pubertal Phase:

Because of puberty and menstruation, ladies are prone to premenstrual stress syndrome which may include bloating, mood changes a few days before menses and gets relieved only when the menses starts. Usually, it is mild. The severe symptoms could be treated with antidepressants.

Pregnancy and childbirth:

Immediately after delivery of a baby, the mother may go through post-partum blues which means feeling low in mood for a few days after delivery. It is only temporary, and it resolves by itself. Sometimes, it can be followed by post-natal depression if the low mood persists for at least two weeks or more. A specialist can treat this kind of depression.

Menopause:

When menopause happens around 45 years of age, there are mood changes, hot flushes, dryness of the vagina, etc., which are usually mild symptoms. Hormone replacement therapy helps in severe cases.

CHAPTER 17

STOPPING SMOKING

Case 21: A middle-aged man smokes cigarettes about two packets a day. He continues to smoke despite health problems.

Answer: Nicotine addiction can be treated with behavioural therapy, counselling, nicotine replacement therapy and a few specific drugs if needed. Early intervention can help to prevent the development of nicotine dependence.

Cigarette smoking is the leading preventable cause of death worldwide. Tobacco contains nicotine and many carcinogens. So, it increases the risk of many acute and chronic diseases, including the risk of cancer in many sites. Millions of smokers are attempting to quit each year. Nicotine withdrawal symptoms often make the process of quitting difficult. In this chapter,

I will tell you how you can come off cigarette-smoking addiction.

What are the effects of nicotine in tobacco?

It boosts mood, produces a sense of wellbeing, enhances concentration and short-term memory. Due to these reasons, smoking can be addictive, and it can also cause dependence.

Benefits of smoking cessation:

+ Reduces the risk of damage to eyes such as cataracts.

+ Decreases chance of having a heart attack, stroke and various cancers like lung cancer, oral cancer, etc.

+ Can add years to one's life.

What are the symptoms of nicotine withdrawal?

The symptoms usually reach a peak in 2-3 days after you quit and are gone within 1-3 months.

Some of the common symptoms include intense cravings for nicotine, anxiety, depression, headache, poor sleep and weight gain.

Management:

The successful intervention begins with identifying users and giving appropriate intervention based upon the patient's willingness to quit.

Five significant steps to intervention are 5 As - Ask, Advise, Assess, Assist and Arrange.

1. *Ask about tobacco use and passive smoking:* Identify high-risk cases like heavy smokers who smoke 25 or more cigarettes a day. Chewing tobacco leads to oral cancer. Passive smoking is breathing in other people's tobacco smoke which is also harmful, and it is as bad as active smoking. Passive smoking can cause premature death in non-smokers.

2. *Advise:* Advise about harmful effects of smoking and emphasize the need to quit smoking.

3. *Assess:* Assess clinically about dependency and severity of drug abuse. The severity of symptoms varies according to the duration and quantity of tobacco used.

4. *Assist:* Assist by discussing various treatment options and by using motivational interviewing to quit and stay off smoking.

5. *Arrange:* Arrange for necessary tests and admission to de-addiction centres when appropriate, which offer detoxification using behavioural therapy, medicines, counselling and supervision.

First-line treatment for smoking cessation is NRT – nicotine replacement therapy, and the use of Varenicline and Bupropion, which are antidepressant medicines.

The aim of the treatment is to decrease symptoms of nicotine withdrawal, making it easier to stop using cigarettes. Patient's preference decides the choice of treatment.

Studies show that NRT is effective for smoking cessation. This can be used for people smoking more than 10 cigarettes per day. It can be a transdermal patch, gum, or lozenge.

Nicotine transdermal patch – long-acting and is simplest to use. Patient compliance is high. Compliance means strictly following the doctor's advice.

Nicotine gum is short-acting, chewable, and available in many flavours.

Nicotine lozenge is a short-acting NRT Product.

Narcotics Anonymous – a non-profit organization is available for support.

In some countries, quit phone line numbers are also available.

In conclusion, the more you try to quit, the more likely you will succeed as help is available within your reach.

CHAPTER 18

AGE RELATED MEMORY LOSS

Case Example 22: A 65-year-old man keeps forgetting the names of even his close friends and could not recognise their faces. This has been happening for the past 6 months and it has been worsening gradually. He could not perform his day-to-day activities due to his memory issues.

Management of this case: This is a case of dementia. Seeing the psychiatrist at an early phase will help in identifying the problem sooner. The doctor will ask a set of simple questions called mini mental state examination and do some tests if needed. Good drugs are available to prevent worsening of the symptoms. Simple memory aids like pocket diary, mind games, regular reading habits, etc. also can help.

Even though memory issues are more common as you age, memory loss is not a part of normal aging.

What is Dementia?

Dementia is memory loss associated with confusion about time, place, person, problems in speaking or writing, wandering behaviour and asking the same questions repeatedly.

This condition occurs in people who have genetic predisposition, diabetes, high blood pressure, alcohol abuse, deficiency of some vitamins and head injury.

Memory loss is very difficult to manage when people live alone. They could endanger their life and others by actions like leaving the gas on in the kitchen, forgetting to lock the doors, etc.

CHAPTER 19

MISCELLANEOUS TOPICS

Case Example 23: A person who has a mental illness did not go for regular follow up as he felt he was better now but the arguments in the family gradually increased over a period of time. He stopped taking his medicines against doctors' advice.

Management of this case: This patient has poor insight into his illness. It is the responsibility of the caretaker to seek help of the care provider or even the law enforcement authorities if needed in order to provide adequate follow up and medications. For any mentally ill patient the information given by the caretaker is very helpful for the doctors to plan their treatment.

Why is mental illness on the rise?

The World Health Organization (WHO) projects that mental disorders are increasing significantly.

Some of the reasons for mental illness are listed below:

+ Increased pressures from parents or society

+ Increased performance pressures (education, career, financial)

+ Poor sleep

+ Increase in sexually explicit material

+ Reduced parental contact and the breakdown of the family unit

+ Reduced face-to-face interactions and social supports

+ Sexual orientation confusion

+ Being exposed to aggressive behaviour

+ Use of recreational drugs

+ Social stigma about mental illness which prevents people from asking for help

+ Screening of mental illnesses not happening prior to marriage.

Caretaker's stress:

People having mental illnesses may or may not suffer due to their condition. However, the caretakers always have difficulty in coping and caring for them when mental illness is present for a prolonged period. Hence, the caretakers also need adequate support and counselling.

Difficulty in Caring for the mentally ill:

Lack of insight in the patient about their illness causes a challenging situation for the caretakers. Patients may refuse regular consultation, and they may avoid taking the drugs regularly.

ANNEXURE: A

Frequently Asked Questions:

1) Can a mentally ill patient recover and lead a normal life at all?

   Yes, Certainly. The degree of recovery depends on the type of illness and the support system available.

---

2) Does the patient need to take medications life long?

   Many drugs can be stopped by the treating doctor after treating for a short course and reassessing the situation. Whereas some patients need these drugs for life.

---

3) Can a mentally ill patient stop taking drugs immediately by himself after starting to feel better?

   Never stop the drugs without consulting the doctor. Usually, doctors continue the drugs for at least 6 months to 1 year after patient has started to feel better, especially in case of drugs for mind.

4) Do these drugs have lots of side effects?

All chemicals do have side effects. But we must weigh the pros and cons and use the drugs appropriately. Usually, doctors prescribe the time-tested safe drugs only. Doctors also warn about any usual side effects that can be expected like dizziness, stomach upset or weight gain.

5) What is the best time to take drugs for the mind – morning or evening?

Some drugs cause drowsiness during daytime affecting the quality of life. Based on that doctor will advise you.

6) Marriage is believed to cure some mental illnesses. Is that true?

It is a myth. Marriage is not a cure. Before marriage try to treat the condition effectively and bring the condition under good control.

7) What is the difference between a psychiatrist and a psychologist?

Psychiatrists are medically qualified doctors, specializing in the treatment, diagnosis, and prevention of mental health problems.

Psychologists specialize in the study of mind and behaviour or in the treatment of mental, emotional, and behavioural disorders.

An important point to be aware is that **Psychiatrists** can prescribe medicine whereas **Psychologists** cannot.

ANNEXURE: B

Sources of help:

(Please find the latest contact numbers on Google)

International Help Lines:

Al Anon - for alcohol abuse

Alcoholics Anonymous - for alcohol abuse

Asian Family Counselling Service

Cruse Bereavement Care

Depression Alliance

Families Anonymous

Weight Watchers club

Home-Start International

Narcotics Anonymous - for substance abuse

Relate - for marital counselling

Samaritans

SANE – Schizophrenia, A National Emergency

SANEline

Indian Help Lines:

SCARF - Schizophrenia Research Foundation, Chennai: +91 44 26151073

The Banyan - for homeless women: +91 9677121099

SNEHA - suicide prevention helpline, Chennai: +91 44 24640050

Apollo ambulance phone number - 1066

Ambulance (Government-State) phone number - 102

Women helpline phone number -1091

Women helpline (domestic abuse) phone number - 181

Recommended YouTube channels:

Dr. Padma's Pearls of Wisdom in English and Tamil

Psychiatrist Pratap - in Tamil and English

Dr. Radhika Kelkar - in Hindi and English

Author's email ID - anbuextra@gmail.com

ANNEXURE: C

Useful info for patients and care takers:

Guidelines for doctor consultation:

1. Choose a professional with the right qualification and work experience.
2. Trust and a good rapport between the doctor and the patient are essential for a reasonable recovery rate.
3. Involve the patient in the decision-making process if possible.
4. Discuss the importance of relapse prevention for a better quality of life in the long term.
5. Use prompts to encourage patients to keep their follow-up appointments.

Guidelines for drug treatment:

1. Use dosette boxes for being organized.
2. Educate patients to encourage compliance with taking medicines.
3. Use medicines with fewer side effects.

4. Keep a simple drug regimen and use only necessary medications.

5. Get family support to monitor the patients for safety and compliance of drug use.

6. Plan and buy medicines in advance before the tablets run out of stock.

7. Medications in this field of mental health do work by correcting the neurochemical imbalance in the brain. These medicines have to be taken for a considerable period, sometimes even for a lifetime, if necessary, in severe cases.

CONCLUSION

It has been a fantastic journey writing this book from the start to finish. Please read the book a few times to fully grasp what is being said.

Living a balanced life is possible only if we have adequate understanding of people around us, having a peaceful mind, willing to compromise, being surrounded by supporting friends and family, eating healthy, doing regular exercise and practising meditation. Also understanding the root cause of the problems we face helps in effectively solving the problems.

Most of the people carry on their life without proper awareness of their thoughts and the thoughts of people around them. That leads to a shallow unhappy life. This book would have given some idea into what is happening in yours as well as in other's mind. This gives courage to face life issues with confidence.

Wishing you a blissful blessed life ahead.

www.ingramcontent.com/pod-product-compliance
Lightning Source LLC
Chambersburg PA
CBHW031318250726
48656CB00005B/1852